Applauding *Exercise Enthusiastically*

I attest to Harriet West Gordon, LPC, commitment to exercise and fitness. My relationship with Mrs. Gordon developed through "A David Dance Company" where students of all ages were taught various art forms of dance while building character. She became a surrogate studio-mom, advocate and intercessor for our students and company. I later learned of her personal love of liturgical dance and had the opportunity to watch her minister on numerous occasions with vibrancy and passion. She embodies the purpose of movement both physically and spiritually. Mrs. Gordon is dedicated to exercising her

"Faith through examples of her "Works." I am grateful that she is transferring her knowledge and passion that will help others.

Ladisa Robinson Onyiliogwu
Co-founder, Entrepreneur
"The GoodLIFE" Company

In life we go from one anxious moment to another. It is imperative that we stop justifying unhealthy lifestyle habits, then search for quick fixes to become healthy. Harriet Gordon, LPC, has written a fascinating handbook which will assist you with your transformation to a healthier you.

Glenn D. Gordon,
B.S. Sociology/Fitness Advocate

Our bodies are not our own; we were bought with a price. So we must be faithful stewards of God's property.

**Madonna Woolford
R.N., B.S.N**.

We need to be proactive in health: Mind, Body, Spirit, and Soul.

**Debra Griffin Stevens
D.N.P., M.S.N., R.N.C-M.N.N.**

Movement is vital to the human spirit. Exercise daily, as you "Go Wild" for Jesus.

**1K Phew (Glenn "Isaac" Gordon, II)
Hip-Hop Artist**

Human expression of righteousness is incomplete unless there is focus on sanctifying the body. I am personally encouraged to make these dictums a permanent part of my life. It is my hope that you will do the same.

AnthonyWilliams
M.D., M.P.H.

HARRIET WEST GORDON

PEEL

EXERCISE ENTHUSIASTICALLY

NO BRANCH CAN BEAR FRUIT BY ITSELF;
IT MUST REMAIN ON THE VINE.
JOHN 15:4B

DISCLAIMER

The information presented herein is in no way intended as a substitute for medical counseling. This book was written to provide experiential information. Neither Harriet West Gordon, or GHD Inc., nor any member of the organization's board shall have liability or responsibility to any person with respect to damage, injury, or any alleged causes resulting from information in this book.

All scripture quotations, unless otherwise indicated, are from the King James Version of the Holy Bible.

RESOURCES

www.stretchingexercisesforbusypeople
www.dancestyles.org
www.carlafields.com

Cover designed by Harriet Gordon, LPC

ISBN: 978-0-9862166-2-6

GOD'S DIVINE HANDWORK, INC.

Our organization's goal is to affect the lives of people in the communities which we serve. God's Divine Handiwork, Inc. (GHDI), is a family-oriented organization which has deep concern for the well-being of our society. We desire to see people "well" in all aspects of their lives. We aim to educate society regarding academic, spiritual, emotional, and physical health. Conferences, forums, seminars, classes, and workshops may be arranged for your specific needs. Our services include courses entitled, but not limited to:

Healthy Living
Test-Taking Tips
Time Management
Parenting to the End
PEEL, Volume 1: *Pray Powerfully*
PEEL, Volume 2: *Eat Efficiently*
PEEL, Volume 3: *Exercise Enthusiastically*
PEEL, Volume 4: *Learn, Laugh, & Live Lovingly*
PEEL, Volume 5: Cook Consciously

Contacts us: **peelv5@gmail.com,**

www.harrietwestgordon.com and on Facebook:

http://www.facebook.com/peelv5

"It's the quality of your days rather than the quantity of your years that really counts.

Enjoy life!"

—Harriet Gordon, LPC

DEDICATION

PEEL, Volume 3: *Exercise Enthusiastically* is dedicated to the Body of Christ who can live victoriously in every area of life – which includes taking care of your total health and fitness.

Dedicated to those who have always given me unconditional love and support:

My Family

CONTENTS

ACKNOWLEDGEMENTS

Thank you for your unconditional love
and support through the years:

*My husband, Glenn; daughter, Dawn
(Jeremiah); son, Glenn "Isaac" and my
extended family.*

www.dancestyles.org

Dawn Gordon Smith, Trainer,
Entrepreneur

www.carlafields.com

Carla Fields, Certified Trainer, Aerobics
Instructor

FOREWORD

$\mathcal{H}$aving a passion for fitness and its benefits is rewarding. Harriet West Gordon, LPC, shares my passion, and enthusiasm for living a healthy lifestyle. Therefore, I am sharing my workout routines, in hopes that others will be encouraged, and inspired then make healthy lifestyle changes.

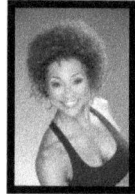

At The Center of my Life is God the father, his son Jesus Christ, always put them First, start each day with Prayer, and Meditation, let go of Stress and things that take you away *from* reaching your goal.

Fitness is my Job, I must Look, Practice, and Teach Fitness. I actually practice and write out each routine on a daily basis. The Routine always changes from week to week. I work out with 2 or 3 workout partners, and we push each other. Fitness is a way of life not something I do when I feel like it. People say it's in my blood I can't help it, I'll always work out, because it makes me feel good about myself. I actually work out harder when I don't have to be stressed out about competition or an event, like say a trade show in which I have to perform. When I'm working out, I like to take my time and focus on me and areas I need improvement. I also meditate a lot, and I get in a zone, and I don't like interruptions. I don't work out to get ready for a competition, I compete because I'm always ready and because it takes me to the next level.

I Superset, Interset, … Go Heavy, then light… mix in drills… Steps, Leaps/Jumps, Bike Spin, Treadmill sprint, with Weight lifting. We hit every body part (Chest, Biceps, Back Shoulders, Quads, Hams, Glutes, Abs-upper/lower/obliques). Personally I work out 2-3 hours a day, usually weights and cardio in the morning for 90 minutes, and in the evenings Corporate Wellness for Kaiser Permanente, or V103. Kick boxing on Saturdays and Stadium stairs. Sometimes I think I'll take a day off and just walk outdoors or play with my son, but it usually turns into something intense… I just feel better when I work out. I drag my clients along, which pushes me and them.

Carla Fields Fitness, Inc.
Phone: 678.283.9978
fax:770.559.3111
5404 Hillandale Park Drive, Suite
B, Lithonia GA 30058
Website: www.carlafields.com
email: carlafields@carlafields.com

PREFACE

---

*F*amilies, pastors, other community leaders, and individuals who desire to empower others and themselves will be blessed by this book. It is impossible to exude healthy nurturing if you are unhealthy. While proper healthcare can break strongholds in geographical regions and individual lives, proper relaxation has been known to calm raging bulls. Compiled in this book are numerous details for well-being. Emails, for example, may represent frustration for some readers.

Figure 1

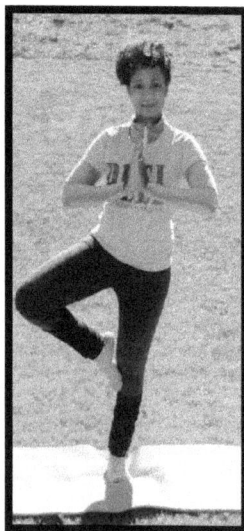

Try this technique:

While you are reading your email, remember to

breathe slowly and focus your attention on your breath. Make the "out" breath two times longer than the "in" breath. This will calm you, immediately.

Breathe

When you want to gain endurance and strength, breathing exercises will empower your mind to remain focused, calm and alert. They will strengthen you physically and help you in multiple ways: aide the skeletal, digestive, immune, and other systems. You may be surprised how powerful these simple stretches really are once you begin to do them with ease throughout the day. Proper breathing is a great contribution to well-being. Additional healthy factors are:

Well-being

- *Sunshine* – 15 minutes in the sun will lower your blood pressure. It also turns your body's cholesterol into Vitamin D. It is free, use it!

- *Water* – Drink lots of it. It will cleanse your body tissues and give you energy.

- *When to Eat* – Eat your largest meal in the morning, a moderate lunch, and sparingly in the evenings. Meals should be spaced 4 to 5 hours apart.

- *When to Drink* – Drink 15 to 20 minutes before meals or two hours after meals. Drink at least 8 glasses of water per day.

- *When to Sleep* – Our bodies heal themselves between 9p.m. and 12 midnight. Every hour of sleep that you get before midnight is worth two hours of sleep that you get after midnight.

This is the third in a series. For victory in every area of your life, consider, along with the consultation from your physician, the advice from each volume of P.E.E.L.

P.   PRAY POWERFULLY – Vol. 1

E.   EAT EFFICIENTLY –   Vol. 2

E.   EXERCISE
      ENTHUSIASTICALLY -Vol. 3

L.   LEARN, LAUGH, LIVE, LEAD
        LOVINGLY   – Vol. 4

"Quality rather than quantity measures time on earth."

CHAPTER 1

EARLY MORNING

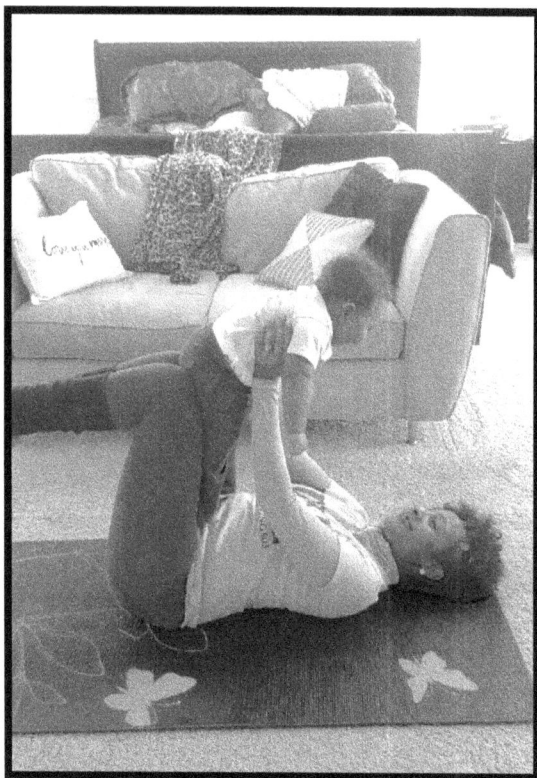

Please consult your physician before engaging in any physical activity. This book includes exercises for men, women, teens, and children. Because of known health challenges, this content takes the most effort to write. However, my intellect tells me that I have come too far to slumber. If you are feeling low before you exercise, you will feel energized by the end.

Schedule breaks. Schedule times during the day, week, month, and year to relax and rejuvenate. Maybe just a five-minute stretch break after each meeting. Remember, treat yourself and your body to regular massages (In one form or another), hot baths, Jacuzzi, or walking. You may get along better with others when you treat yourself better, and you are most productive.

A wonderful benefit to exercise is improved sleep habits. Physical activity will ensure that your body and mind are ready for a great night's sleep. It promotes better energy levels. It may sound unlikely, but the more you exercise, the more energy you will have. Bothersome chores will feel much easier, and you will be able to do more for longer periods of time.

Another benefit is decreasing stress levels. Worries tend to diminish in size while you are concentrating on working out. You will feel more in control of yourself and your life. It can improve self-esteem and self-confidence. Exercising regularly, improves circulation throughout the body. I have witnessed the improved circulation resulting in a glowing complexion and improved transportation of oxygen around my body. Some healthy tips to emphasize are:

Preventive Check Ups

If you have a concern about your health, it is important to get it checked out before it becomes a problem. Regular

Figure 2

checkups will ensure that your physician and you are working toward the same goal – your best health! Additionally, maintain a current "To –Do" List, daily. Clean out clutter; mess can equal stress.

Physical Activity

Joining a club may prove beneficial; such as, a dance group, bike club, sports team, walkers, runners, or a gym. Choose an activity that you enjoy. Thirty minutes a day may change your life. There are activities you may do during your regular day to day routine: **Stand Straight/Sit Straight** – slouching may cause the brain to receive less oxygen. **Stretch** – stand on your toes and extend your palms to the ceiling. **Breathe** – just a few deep breaths get the oxygen moving through your system.

See the exercises below, some fit best with your morning routine. Try them to find out which fit best:

Keen Hearing

Sit up in bed and breathe gently into your belly. Feel your body soften and your mind relax. Focus on the days' activities. Think about what you want to accomplish and what the day will bring. Breathe deeply.

Do you want to pay closer attention? "Sweaty Exercise" helps the thinking process (Excuse the pun). If you are in search of a treatment that does not require medicine; look no further. Exercise.

Consequently, what you eat may effect your thinking. Eating foods high in Omega-3 fatty acid, like salmon, encourages new cell growth.

Power Smoothie

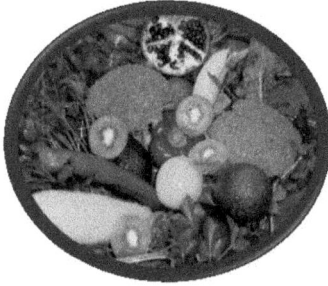

Figure 3

Feed your mind and your body. Gather ingredients then mix together in a blender.

Measure amounts as you prefer until you get desired consistency:
Almond or Soy Milk
Fruit Juice
Berries (may be frozen)
1 Banana
Spinach
Whey or Soy Protein Powder
Be creative and include other ingredients.

(Read "PEEL EAT EFFICIENTLY" by Harriet Gordon, LPC)

Hand Calisthenics

As often as possible, stretch your hands and wrists:
Move hands in all directions and stretch, with hands in a prayer position.
Squeeze fists tightly.
Stretch fingers wide.
Interface fingers and stretch up.

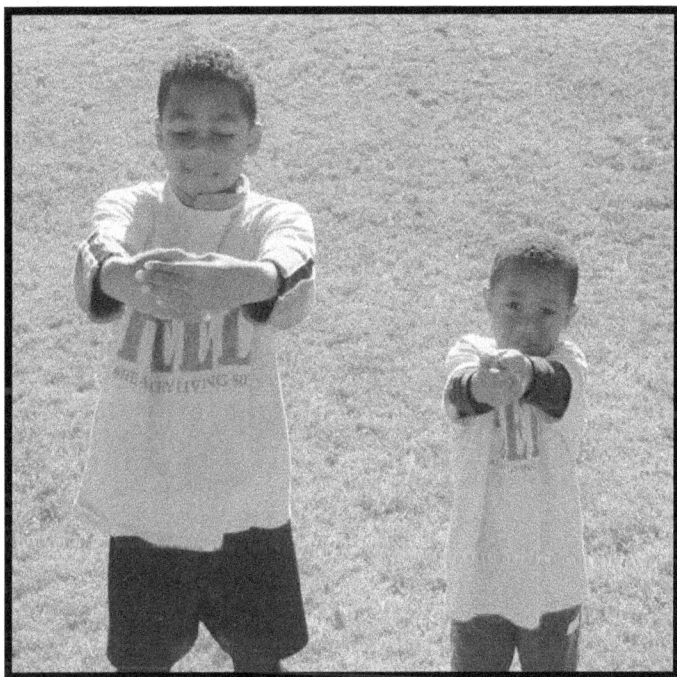

Figure 4

Rise and Shine

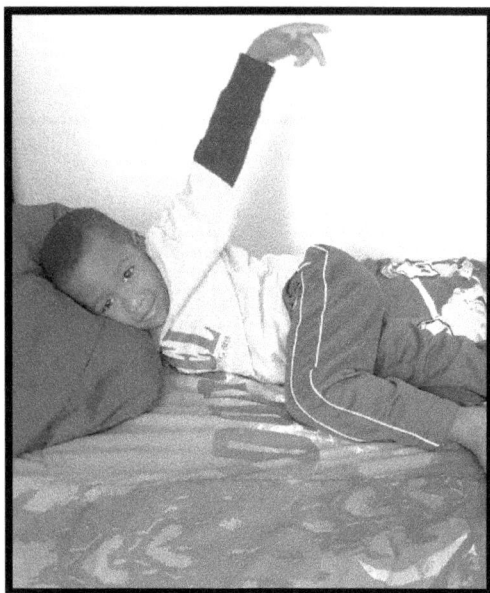

Figure 5

Sit up in bed and breathe.
Feel your body soften and your mind relax,
Focus on the day's activities.
Think about what you want to accomplish
And what the day will bring. Breathe
deeply.

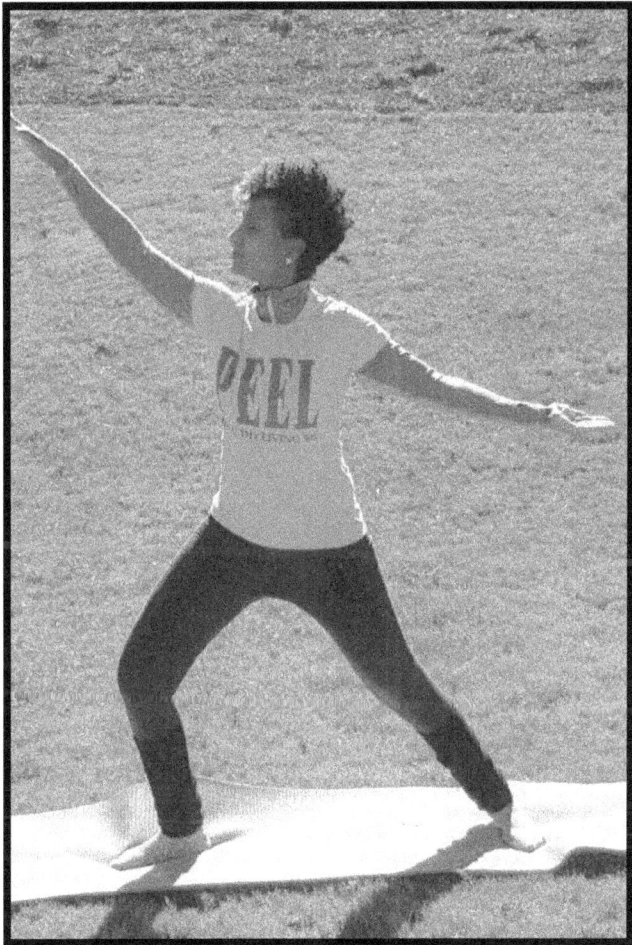

Figure 6 *Warrior Pose*

Warrior Pose

Raise your arms to the side with fingers pointed.

Take a big step to the side; with your right foot turned to the side and knee bent.

Keep your left foot planted, your leg straight.

Your upper body should be straight and strong; shoulders relaxed.

Do not hold your breath!

Relax into the stretch, then gently release.

Return to a standing position.

Switch sides, then repeat.

The Facedown

Lean facedown over a table.

Keep feet on or near the floor.

Comfortably breathe and relax.

Feel your whole body weight resting on the table.

(Be gentle with your lower back)

A towel or pillow may be used under your midsection.

Take your time and relax into the stretch

<u>Morning Run</u> - Time to get outdoors and enjoy nature. Whether you walk briskly, jog, or run, be sure that you extend your legs and arms as *intentional* motions. Exercise your muscles and tendons to give motion to your joints.

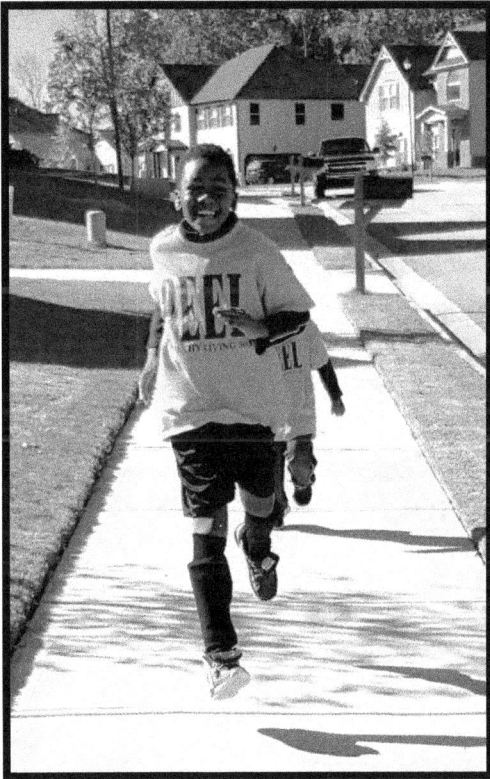

Figure 7   **Morning Run**

Self – Massage

Place both hands on your shoulders and neck.
Squeeze both hands and palms.
Rub vigorously.
Keep shoulders relaxed.
Wrap one hand around the other forearm.
Squeeze the muscles with thumbs and fingers.
Move up and down from your elbow to fingertips and back.
Repeat.

"Treat yourself and your body to massages, regularly."

CHAPTER 2

DAY TIME

Over 60 percent of workplace ailments are represented by repetitive strain injuries. They may be cured with early diagnosis. See a physician if you have constant pain in the hands, wrists, or forearms. As a professional, I am in regular (sometimes more) use of keyboards. Often, daily tasks become difficult with stiffness and swelling. My therapist diagnosed me as having Carpal Tunnel and prescribed a range of exercises.

Complete these exercises, daily, to avoid wearing the "glamorous" brace which I remember adding to my wardrobe:

1. Place one forearm on a table on a towel for padding with one hand off the edge of the table.
Move your hand until you feel a stretch.

2. Stand or sit with your arm at your side with the elbow bent to 90 degrees, palm down.
3. Begin with your thumb positioned out. Move the thumb across the palm and back.

A good tip to remember is drink lots of water whenever you feel tired. Fatigue is a common symptom of dehydration. Here are some simple stretch exercises recommended for day time use:

Kick Back Log-On Pose

Interlace your fingers behind your head.
Relax your elbows and shoulders.
Smile, breathe, and stretch your elbows back.
Let the tightness release, slowly.
Repeat throughout the day.

Human Basketball Net

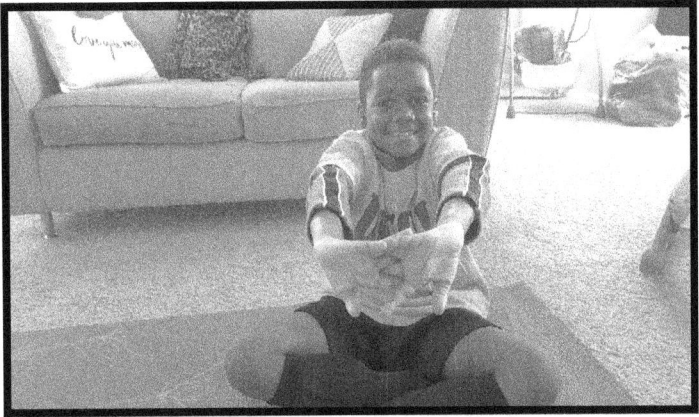

Figure 8

Raise your arms straight above your head.
Interlace your fingers.
Alternate palms upward and downward.
Stretch your arms out in front and relax
your shoulders.

Reaching Hands

Hold your arms out to the side.
Stretch with your fingertips to the opposite
walls.

Breathe and relax.
Arms outstretched.
Slowly tilt sideways as a windmill.
Reach for the ceiling and the floor.
Gently stretch the midsection.
Return to a seated position.
Breathe and relax.

Chest Stretch

Seated on the edge of the chair.
Hold the sides of the seat.
Gently stretch up and forward.
Open your chest and tilt your head back.
Relax and breathe into the stretch.

Feet and Ankles

As you talk on the phone, stretch your legs and
Rotate your ankles and feet.
Notice your attention increase as you stretch.

Headache Solution

Place your index fingers in the middle and just above each eyebrow, press with your fingers, and hold. Close your eyes and breathe deeply.

Eye Strain Solution

Take mini breaks from your computer screen as you work. Every ten minutes, refocus and look around the room instead of the screen. Each hour, close your eyes. Slowly roll your eyes. Take a few breathes and return to your work.

Balance Tree Pose- Figure 9

(To minimize nervousness or stress)
Remove shoes and stand next to a table or chair for balance.
Raise your right foot against the inside of your thigh.

Place your right hand on your right foot if it slides down.

If you feel steady, place your hands by your chest in a prayer position.

Feel the standing foot rooted into the ground.

Relax and breathe.

Stand straight and balanced.

Switch legs slowly.

Elevator Stretch

Place your right hand on the wall facing you.

Stand straight and bend your left leg back.

With your left hand, hold your toes and pull your foot

To your buttocks.

Breathe, hold, release, switch sides.

Repeat.

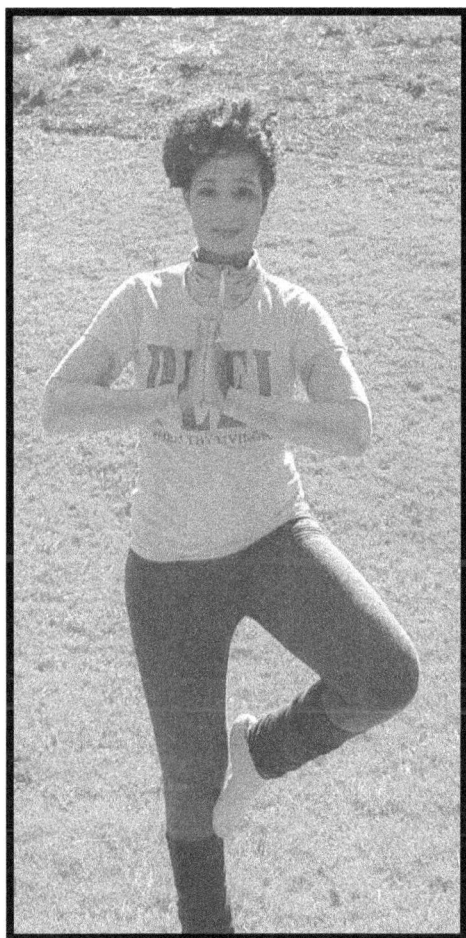

Figure 9 Balance Tree Pose

Copier Stretch

Place your hands on the edge of the copier.
Stand with the feet apart.
Drop your head to chest.
Breathe and relax your shoulders.

You Got This Stretch!

While seated, cross left leg over right.
Place right hand or elbow on the crossed knee.
Gently turn your body left and look behind you.
Switch legs, twist in opposite direction.
Repeat.

"Fatigue is a common symptom of dehydration."

CHAPTER 3

MIDDAY – LUNCH

When you eat nutritiously, you feel better. Take time out to eat during your lunch break; not work.

Tips:

- ✓ Snack on fruit or nuts only when you are hungry.
- ✓ Order a salad with your meal.
- ✓ Eat light.
- ✓ Skip quick fixes; as sugar and caffeine.
- ✓ Drink herbal teas.

What do you think will happen to body cells without motion? The body needs physical activity because the tissue cells, of which the body is composed require daily stimulation to maintain their elasticity. Cells will stop functioning if they continue to go without exercise. They will become weak and begin to malfunction if they are not exercised on a regular basis. Without motion, the body cells will slowly die. When you exercise vigorously on a regular basis, you will experience fewer health problems than a person who does not exercise. Additionally, a person who exercises removes the toxins and debris from their system. When the body does not receive a sufficient supply of oxygen people become forgetful.

The most important muscle to exercise is the heart muscle. When the heart is not exercised, it starts to function improperly, arteries clog, strokes and heart attacks may result. When an unexercised heart is suddenly exerted, it may be fatal. Mowing the lawn with force and shoveling snow when the heart muscle has not been exercised are two examples which may cause sudden exertion. Be sure to exercise regularly before engaging in either activity.

Often times, the most powerful exercises are the easiest.

Try these common stretches:

Knee to Chest

Interlace fingers or arms around bent knees.
Gently stretch your knees to chest.
Keeping your hips on the floor.
Hold the stretch.
Breathe into your lower back.
Relax your body, and rest in the pose.

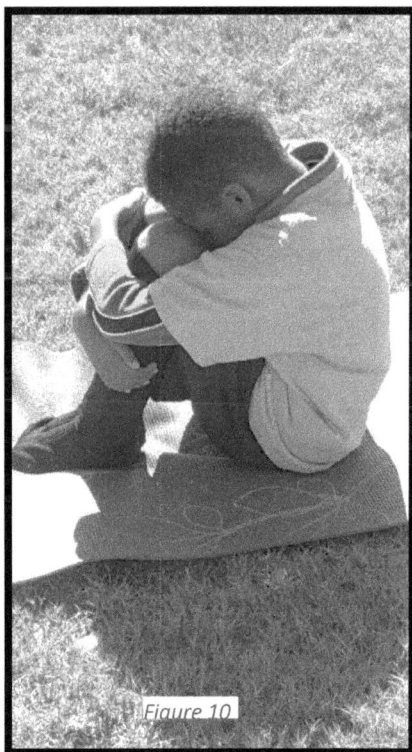

Figure 10

Relaxing the Lower Back

Sit on calves and lay upper body on legs.
Place arms at your side.

Turn face to one side or lay forehead on floor.
Let your body relax and breathe.

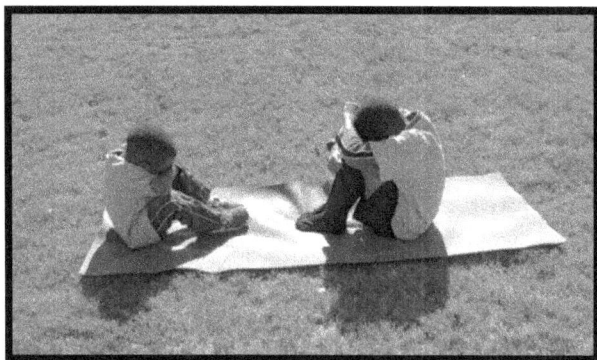

Figure 11

Hands Behind Back

Interlace your fingers behind your back.
Gently bend forward.
Stretch your hands and arms up and back.
Breathe into the stretch.
Gently release arms.
With fists, tap lower back and legs.

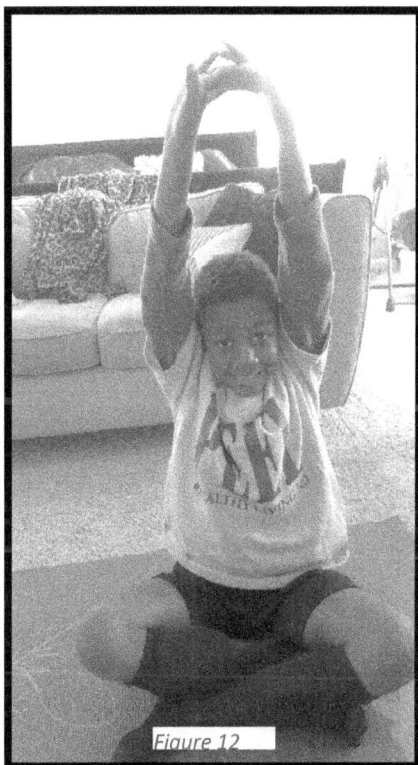

Figure 12

Stretching on the Go

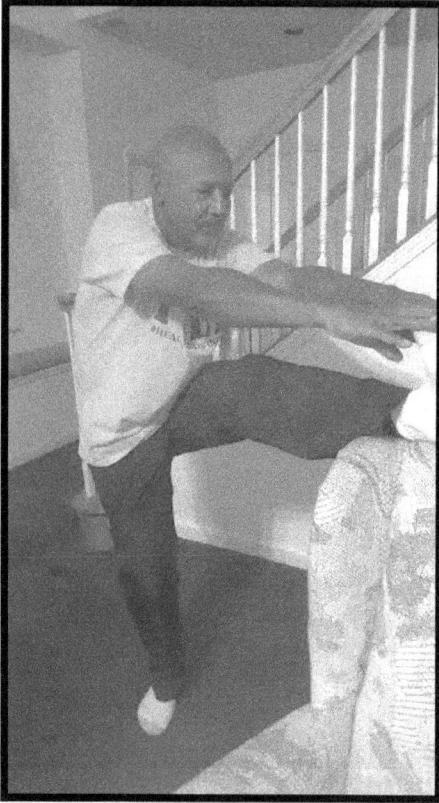

Lift your right foot onto a solid desk or table. Turn your left foot to the side for balance. Stretch over your leg, placing your hands on your leg and

Figure 13

Breathe into the stretch.
Relax your head. Breathe into the stretch.
Flex your foot – breathe.
Switch legs; and repeat.

Power Leg Bends

Place your hand on a solid chair to steady yourself.
Keep your back straight; bend your knees.
Lower your body, slowly, then raise up.
Do this several times, breathing in rhythm.
Try this with your feet flat or heels raised.

"Without motion the body cells will slowly die."

CHAPTER 4

AFTERNOON

$\mathcal{P}$ositive Emotions

Exercise balances emotions. Physical health is extremely important but it is very

Figure 14

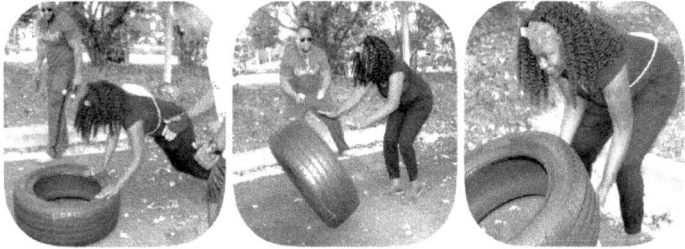

important that we do not neglect our emotional health. It has been proven that exercise aids in the prevention of depression. Emotional problems are sicknesses that many deny. When they are recognized, it is often the symptom rather than the cause that is addressed. How many happy, vibrant people do you know? Feelings stimulated by the mental or physical parts of our body are our emotions. If we were to keep track of one another's emotions and placed them in two columns, one column would outweigh the other. Our emotions deeply affect our lives and the lives of those around us.

It is hard to discern which occurs first: The positive emotion producing a healthy body, or a healthy body
producing a positive mind. A healthy body has a positive effect on our whole being.

When we feel joy, love, happiness, peace, or contentment, there is a surge of pleasure throughout the body and it flows to those around us

Use exercise to keep this surge flowing through your body. When jogging, remember to relax as you exercise. Keep your back straight and your arms and shoulders loose. Shake out your hands and feel your chest stretching out as you breathe deeply. Try these:

Rejuvenation (Vehicle Passenger)

Sit back, relax, and gently roll your head in circles.
Shrug your shoulders up and down, breathing in rhythm
as you shrug.

Stop and Go!

In traffic, loosen your windpipes and sing your favorite song. Imitate an opera singer and come from your belly with the sound.

1,2,3 Kick

Standing in front of a desk with an open space behind you, steady yourself with both hands.
Kick your right leg back with the knee slightly bent.

Stretch and take a deep breath while slowly dropping your leg to the floor.
Switch legs. Repeat

Turn to the side and stretch right leg out.
Relax your body and keep left leg strong; body straight.
Switch sides. Repeat.

Cat Stretch

Raise your head up; arch lower back down.
Exhale as you drop your head, and arch lower back up.
Move slowly; stretch deeply.
Repeat.

Back Stretch – 1

On your back
Bend legs and cross arms over chest.
Breathe deeply and slowly sit halfway up.
Pause. Feeling your belly tighten.
Breathe, release, rest, and Repeat..

Back Stretch – 2

On your back
Bend legs, and at your side and palms down.
Gently stretch your hips.
Breathe, release, and repeat.

There are many benefits for doing Back Stretches. Here are a few:

- ✓ Relax your back and reduce pain.
- ✓ Increase flexibility.
- ✓ Build strength.
- ✓ Reduce risk of back injury.

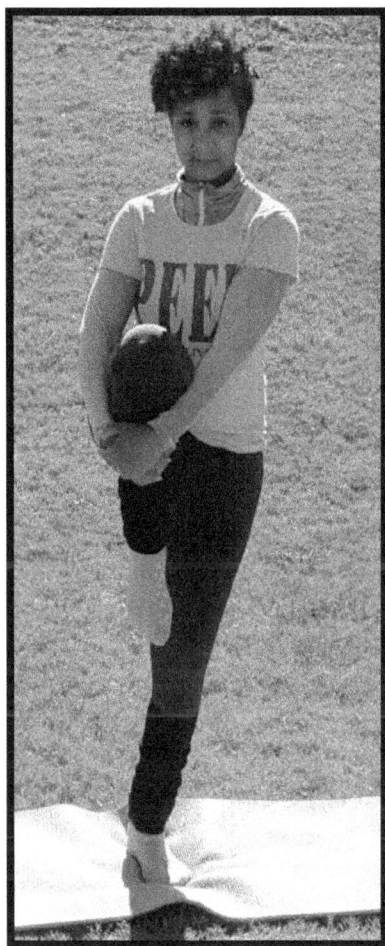

Figure 15 *Body Twist*

Body Twist

Pull right knee to your chest.
Take a deep breath and gently bend your right knee over your left leg.
Hold your right knee down with your left hand over the knee.
Turn your head in the opposite direction.
Take deep gentle breaths and relax your whole body.
Keep both shoulders down.
Gently release, then switch legs.

Power Walk

Walk vigorously for ten minutes.
Focus on breathing.
Take walks outside and observe nature as an added benefit.

Let It GO!

While sitting, reach your hands toward the sky;
Breathe in deeply then relax completely on the exhale.

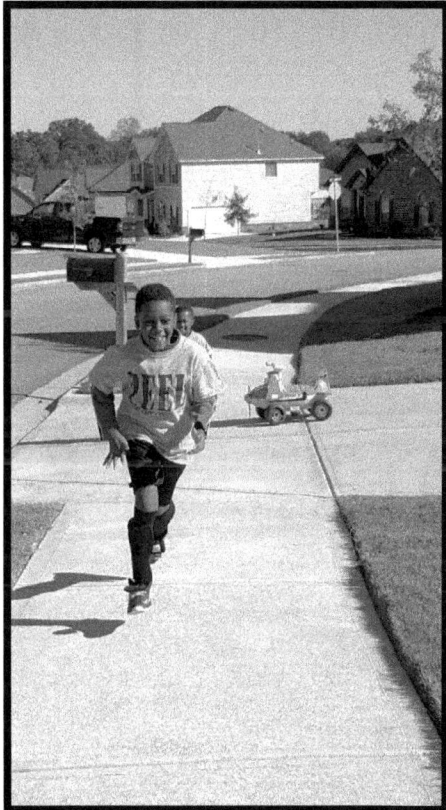

Figure 16 Power Walking

Drop your arms and upper body toward the ground – as a rag doll. (Get ready for this):

While sitting, take the deepest breath and "ROAR" as loudly as you can. Come from your belly with the sound, and open your mouth as wide as you can.

Home! Figure 17

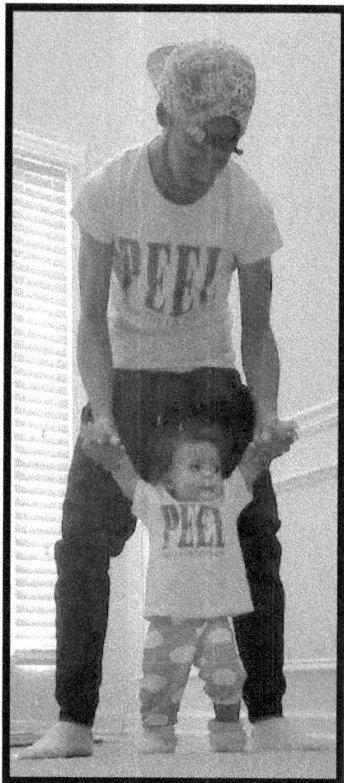

Figure 17 Home!

Free Style – Put on your favorite music, and   for 3 to 5 minutes, twist, shout, dance your body down.   Free style dance and stretch. Focus on releasing the day and just chillax.

Chillaxing

Lie on your back for 3 to 5 minutes and let your thoughts go. Get comfortable by placing a pillow under your knees. Take easy breaths. This will relax the tight spots, calm your mind, and
bring peace.

"Let it go!"

CHAPTER 5

EVENING

Negative Emotions

Negative emotions take energy from the body and hinder the body from cleansing and healing itself. Stress produces more negative emotions when the body is not able to cleanse itself. A person experiences negative emotions when his or her body does not function properly; whether it is due to lack of exercise, a headache, cold, etc. Some emotions send strong waves throughout the body. The emotions of fear, worry, sorrow, hate, jealousy, or anger send negative vibes to others.

Children need plenty of exercise. This may come in the form of music, rhythm, rhyme, rap, drama, charades, role-play, or dance. However, children require more

than occasional exercise. Children have bodies that are hungry
for exercise, because man was created for physical activity. I am in awe when many continue to question, "Why do we exercise?" We exercise because the body cannot function properly without it.

After arriving home and changing into more comfortable clothing; perhaps sweats; complete these relaxation exercises:

Garden of Eden

On your stomach with forearms on the floor.
Keep your elbows beneath your shoulders, slightly supporting your raised upper body.
Keep your hips on the ground and your buttocks tight to support your lower back.
Gently lift your head and chest.
Breathe and stretch, letting the tight areas release.
Hold and breathe.

When you are ready, gently lower yourself to the floor.
Repeat.

Quiet Spot

Find the hidden spot near a chair or a wall.
Lay on your lack and put your legs up.
Breathe.

Bath Time

To relax and renew, treat yourself to a middle of the day mini spa.
Run a hot tub, soft music, candles, oils and bath salts.
Run a hot tube, soft, music soft salts.

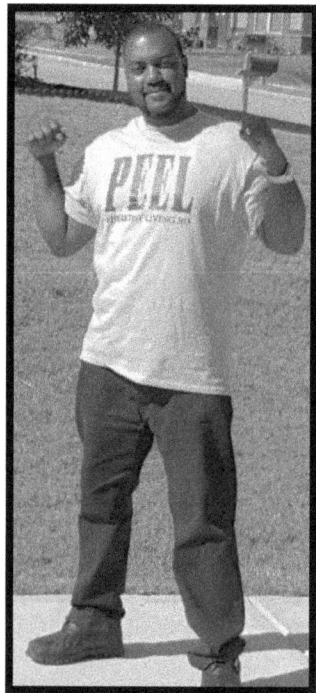

Figure 18 Modified Arm Flex

<u>Couch Potato – or </u>while reading the papers:

Sit on the floor.
Stretch your legs out straight and wide apart.
Slowly walk your hands down your legs.
Gently raise your chest up.
Take a few breaths, then drop your head and shoulders down.
Breathe and relax.

<u>Hot Bath</u>

Relax and renew! Treat yourself to a mini-spa night.
Run a hot tub, put on some soft music, light candles. Use bath oils and salts.

Meditation

While sitting up, place one hand on your belly.
Breathe slowly and deeply.
Feel your hand rise and fall.
Let your shoulders drop.
Feel your body relax and renew.

My favorite and most often used form of meditation is prayer. This is an exercise, though spiritual in nature, medical studies report repeatedly of its benefits to the healing process. This is a form of meditation that I highly recommend.

(Read "PEEL Pray Powerfully" by Harriet Gordon, LPC).

Nighty-night!

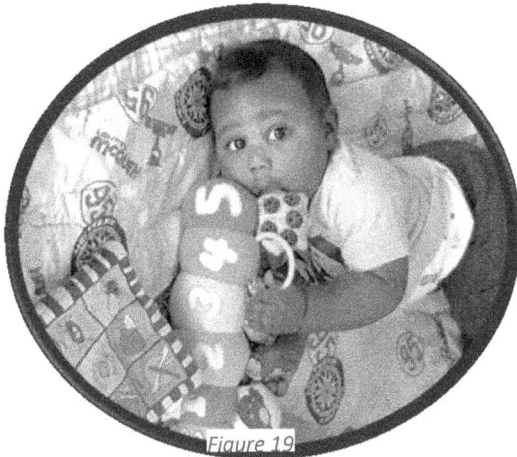

Figure 19

Play soft music or nature sounds. Meditate. Drink herbal tea.

It is my prayer that you are in a more relaxed state than you were before beginning these exercises.

Abundant blessings is my prayer for your life.

"Negative emotions take energy from the body."

CHAPTER 6

CONCLUSION

*T*o enjoy the relaxed feeling that stretching provides, give it an opportunity to work for you. These exercises are natural fits for home or work. When you want to improve or maintain your alertness and physical health, try these exercises and bring serenity to what could be a hectic day.

Tips:

✓ When extending deeply into a stretch, breathe then relax into it. Do not force the stretch.-

✓ When stretching, do not hold your breath. Breathe deeply and slowly, in rhythm with your movements.

✓ If a stretch hurts, do not do it, In other words: "If pain, no gain."

✓ Do one or two stretches fully rather than rushing through many.

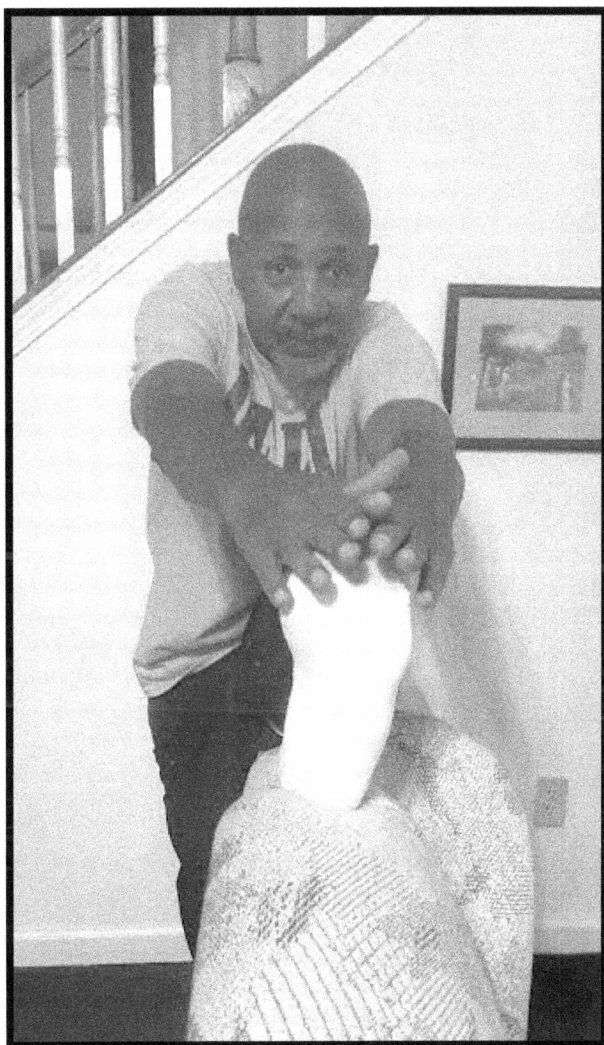

Figure 20 *Stretching*

Exercise Your Way to Excellent Health

ERASE - Erase all mental resistance to the operation of God's power in you. See yourself as a harmonious whole, with mind, body, and spirit working together in harmonious perfection. Hold that mental picture strongly.

ESTABLISH - God creates and he also recreates. Constant establishing is inherent in your being. Therefore, think establishing thoughts about yourself; that you are not running down, but are ever being established.

EXECUTE THE GOD PRINCIPLE - Remember that all health comes from God: health of mind, health of soul, and health of body. Execute the principle in the Biblical statement, "In Him we live, and move, and have our being" (Acts 17:28)

ABOUT THE AUTHOR

HARRIET WEST GORDON

Is an anointed teacher who is dedicated to a *lifetime* of serving. She has passionately and successfully served in ministry roles helping

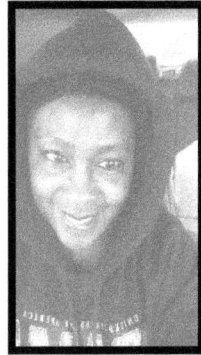

After her morning run

others for over 35 years. September of 1978, she married her college sweetheart, and they are honored parents of two gifted off springs: Glenn "Isaac" Gordon (Hip Hop Artist; Writer-Producer), and Dawn Gordon Smith (Choreographer-Dancer; Teacher).

Harriet adores family life and nature. As a fitness enthusiast, she takes full advantage of her gym membership where she encourages others. She is an education advocate who has received numerous awards for designing and leading transformational train-the-trainer developmental practices. As an *Intentional* Chief Intercessor, she advises parents, youth, young adults, and other intercessors. She gives and donates extra time in areas of research on Aging, Attention Deficit Hyperactivity Disorder (ADHD), Teen Violence, Cancer Awareness, and various intervention / prevention studies. Harriet's passion for family and all humanity leads her to *work* as a sworn

Voters' Registrar. She holds certified licenses in three professions: as a Georgia *Ordained Minister, Counselor, and Teacher.*

As a triple threat, Harriet engages in spiritual warfare on a daily basis. #Sheiswinning!

For appearances, contact:
www.harrietwestgordon.com
or peelv5@gmail.com